PU-ERH-TEE – THE EMPEROR'S TEA

LOWER CHOLESTEROL, BURN FAT, REDUCE CARDIAC AND CIRCULATORY PROBLEMS, DEAL WITH DIABETES: APPLICATIONS OF PU-ERH-TEA IN ITS HOMELAND CHINA

PETER CARL SIMONS

Contents

Preface

Dear reader,

when dealing with natural medicine and alternative healing methods, sometimes it is hard to resist the resurgence of anger.

Recently articles went through the press around the world reporting on "trolls", which had been paid for by the Russian government. According to the report, they were hired to deliberately discredit in blogs and online portals people who were critical of the current Russian Government and its policy.

This type of propaganda is not a modern Russian invention. In fact, the pharmaceutical lobby takes a similar approach. Driven by business interest, it talks bad about products, which have often successfully been used for centuries, even thousands of years, against various ailments. Or they warn based, on an intolerance that could occur every one in a millions of cases, the whole humanity against the product.

Have you ever read the patient information of one of the drugs that these companies sell with the state's blessing? Do it and then decide for yourself whether a natural product could not possibly be an interesting alternative.

It is also always important: If you are writing as an expert on such products, you may under no circumstances make promises of salvation and anyone you advise to use the respective products.

I do not do both because it is true: For taking any preparation plants (as well as for any pharmaceutical product), anyone can promise a cure. Even the best drugs at a certain percentage of users will not have effects - that's not different at all with things from nature. And as with any drug from a pharmacy or drug store, you should take any herbal drug only in consultation with a specialist.

Anyway. Pu-erh tea is a natural product, a freely available tea, which you drink and enjoy like any other over the counter tea. And it is entirely up to you whether you drink pu-erh tea, because if you want to achieve a health effect, it is only a nice side effect while you enjoy its wonderful taste.

In China, its homeland, many people are doing this in any case. With a lot of joy and gratitude, they report positive impacts on their health; even overweight is said to be reduced by the tea. Thought logically there is no reason to assume that the effect of a plant is different, simply because the person, who takes of them, speaks a different language, or was born in another country.

I wish you many hours of pleasure while drinking tea. Similarly, if you experience a positive health effect, contrary to the warnings of certain circles, companies, and associations, don't let the "trolls" hear about it. Instead, quietly look forward to it.

Your Peter Carl Simons

ONE
PU-ERH TEA

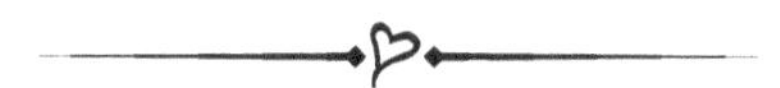

Pu-erh tea is considered by experts as one of the most valuable teas for human health. In China, it has been known for a long time and has been successfully used for the relief of various symptoms, especially in the traditional Chinese medicine.

Renowned scientists are studying at different universities the potency of the Pu-erh teas and their range of applications, sometimes for decades. Known experts are even convinced that we are just beginning with the findings on the application range of this plant.

The often blatant statements of certain circles that pu-erh tea constitutes a panacea and help against anything and everything are still not solid. So you're doing a disservice to the users and only play the "trolls" in their hands.

When looking at the tea, it must be always kept in mind that the most in the western world offered Pu-Erh teas are of extremely poor quality. In China, tea is offered in a variety of quality levels. However, even some well-known European suppliers offer it in such a low quality that it would not be sold in China.

If one intense look around in the market, you will find that tea often corresponds to a price of less than 30 euros per 100 grams of a lower quality level. The effect of tea - but also its taste - is rather low. Really high-quality teas are often traded at various multiples of this price.

TWO

YUNNAN – HOME TO ABOUT 90 PERCENT OF CHINESE HERBAL MEDICINES

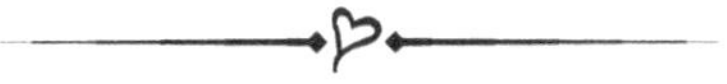

The Yunnan province is also called the "medicinal garden of China". Experts estimate that around 90 percent of the plants that are used today in traditional Chinese medicine originated in this province have which lies in the southwest of China. This eighth largest province of the "Middle Kingdom" is bordered on the north by the province of Sichuan and Tibet in the west and south by Vietnam, Laos and Myanmar.

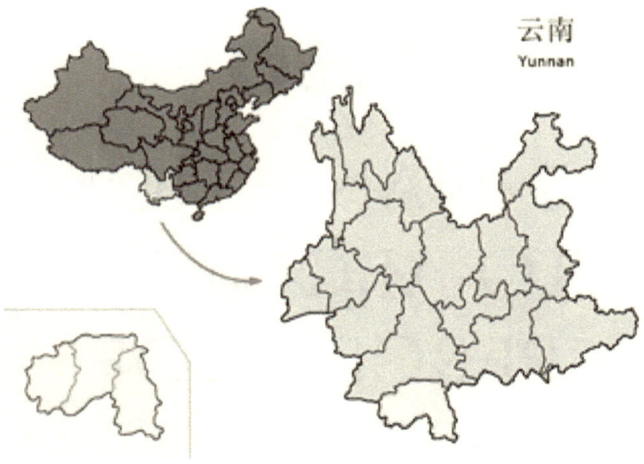

Poetically, the area is also called the "white cloud" or "The Province of Eternal Spring". It includes climatic regions of the tropics to cold alpine zones up to 6740 meters above sea level, such as on Mount Kawagarbo.

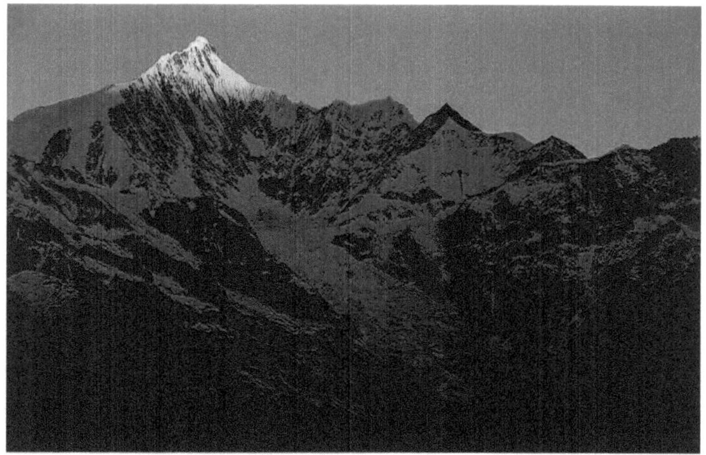

Under the influence of monsoon winds prevails in the Yunnan Province a great climate diversity. So it may happen that all weather conditions from tropical heat to snow occur at the same time in a relatively small area. Such extremes of course also have an impact on the nature and plants.

The variety of the local micro-climate regions makes it possible that a plant paradise with some 20,000 species grows in this area. This is much more than anywhere else in the world - of course, based on a comparable area. No wonder that the region has been described by one "dry scientist" as the "Kingdom of Plants". Due to the relatively large geographic distance from the population centers pollution and commercial overexploitation are fortunately still very limited.

Even historical sources say that the pu-erh tea traditionally comes from six Tea mountains with the names

Youle, Gedeng, Qibang, Mangzhi, Manche, and Manrui. This covers an area of approximately 400 square kilometers, roughly the size of the German federal state of Bremen, or less than half of Rügen.

THREE

THE EMPEROR'S TEA – TODAY FOR ANYONE

The cultivation of Pu-Ehr teas has a long history in Yunnan. Already at the time of the Han Dynasty about 1,700 years ago, the Dai-people produced the tea in the Yunnan Province. The nation is one of more than 80 minorities.

The Chinese medical practitioner Dr. Li Wu cited in his book the Tianhai Yuheng Zhi Tan Cui as follows:

The king of tea trees grows in the tea mountain. He is larger than those of the other five tea mountains and was cultivated by Prince Wu. To date, the locals cherish him by organizing sacrificial ceremonies.

Said Prince Wu was a famous military leader and imperial advisor during the Three Kingdoms period in the year 225. It is reported that the prince - full name Zhuge Liang (181-234) - pushed a campaign in the south forward, where the soldiers began to suffer a mysterious illness. When the Prince inspected the accommodation of his sick soldiers, he pushed his cane into the ground. The stick hit from and grew up a tree. Zhuge Liang plucked the leaves and brewed it into a tea which was instilled by the sick and healed them in no time.

In the autonomous district Xishuangbanna, the southernmost tip of Yunnan, derivatives of the king tree can still be found, and can be about 2000 years old and up to 30 feet tall.

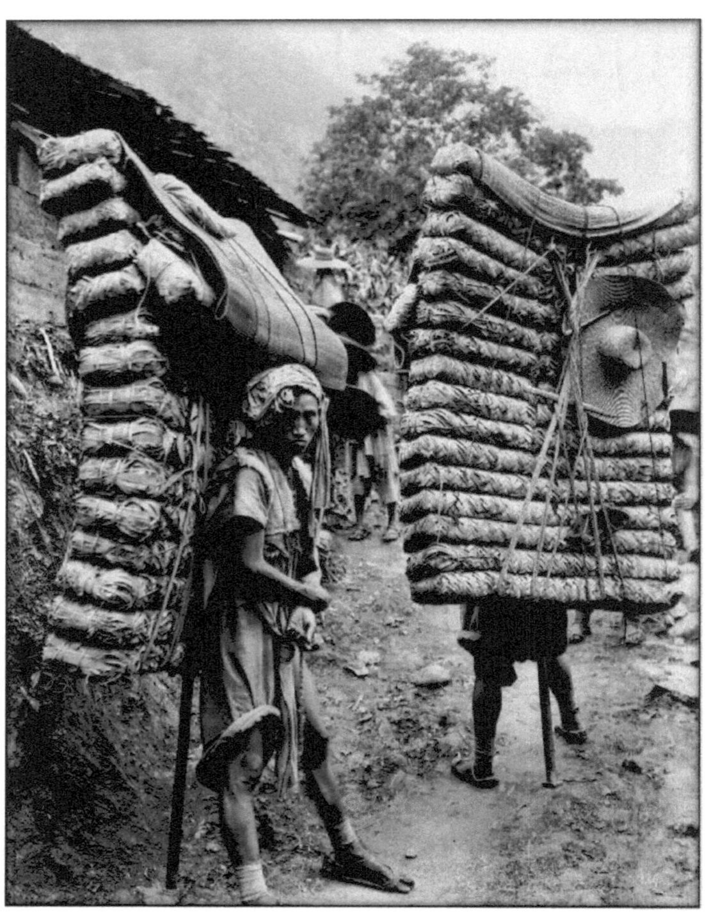

Already in sources from the Tang Dynasty (618-907) it is reported that pu-erh tea was consumed in China's western regions.

In the Song Dynasty (960-1279) the pu-erh tea had a such great importance that it could be used as exchange against a horse and comparable expensive goods.

Later in the Yuan Dynasty (1279-1368), the pu-erh tea eventually became a precious commodity, which was valued among the different population groups in China.

In the Ming Dynasty (1368-1644) the pu-erh tea came along the Silk Road in areas outside of the realm. According to the sources, they offered it in the ball or brick shape that is common today. Sources show that the tea was well known even then in Burma, Thailand, Vietnam and Indonesia and was traded in other countries. During this time, he took his place at the forefront of Chinese teas and gave him since not from.

An idea of the economic significance of tea like a source from 1661, give, wherein it was reported that alone more than 1,500 tons of tea were transported to Tibet annually. Chinese Premier Zhang Hong reported in 1755 according to Dr. Li Wu:

The Pu-tea is a treasure. There are varieties Maojian (Journal prime tea), Yacha (bud tea) and Nii-he (caughter's tea). Maojian is not formed before the year section Guyu (cereals rain), so picked in spring and balls. Its flavor is mild, and he has the scent of lotus. The color is pale green and lovely. The leaves of the Yacha (bud teas) are slightly larger than that of the Maojian, they are formed into spheres which have a weight of two or four have Liang (a Liang corresponds to 30 grams). The population of Yunann appreciates this tea. The daughter's tea (Nü-er cha) is another type of bud tea. It is harvested after the rains and pressed in corn balls between one and ten Jin Jin (a Jin is about 500 grams). What remains after that is coarse and worthless. Chance of these poor quality in Yunnan will be offered. From the very coarse tea leaves is obtained an extract which is thickened and formed into cakes, which you then stamp them. "

Pu Erh was therefore already then formed into cakes or balls of various sizes. Here (hence the name „head tea) are provided the finest tea in head big cake as a tribute to the imperial court. It always consisted of the tenderest buds that had already been rejected during the harvest and were reserved under the threat of punishment for the nobility at the imperial court.

The introduction of protective tariffs by the colonial powers and through the turmoil of the period after the Second World War the tea sales broke down massively. After all, it was about 150 tonnes, ten percent of what had been a few centuries earlier delivered alone from Tibet. Only since the last decades international sales and production volumes increase gradually.

The emperor's tea, also called palace tea of which only about one ton per year is produced, has outlasted the empire. Nevertheless, he continues to be made exclusively of the tenderest leaves of ancient tea trees in complete handmade. Today's Communist government presented this tea selected state visitors as a gift. Presumably, these guests are not even aware what a treasure they get it. At Kaiser times, people were executed already for touching this tea.

FOUR

PREPARATION OF THE TEA

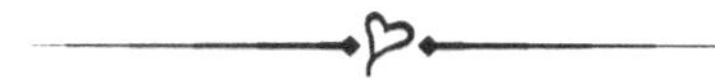

The preparation of the tea takes place in several stages. First, the leaves are harvested and given to wither in a special boiler. Now the workers sort the tea leaves again and free them from foreign matter such as stalks or soil pieces. Depending on the desired level of quality, the tea leaves are then divided and then placed in layers in an absorber, where they are for twenty minutes. Then they come in cloth bag where they are kneaded into brick shapes. The cake thus produced is now stored in a dry place. They are dried in air and finally packaged.

Pu-erh tea is produced in 11 grades, which 10 can be found in stores. The teas differ in terms of their taste, their healing effects and the age of the plants. Often reach inferior, unpressed teas in the European market as well as products of the lower classes. However, teas of classes 6 to 10 are inadvisable unclassified goods. These are sometimes made of rests and are likely to be quite questionable in their effect.

FIVE

SCIENTIFIC RESEARCH

In contrast to German-speaking Europe, where hardly any research results for pu-erh tea is published, the tea is thoroughly investigated in other countries. Dr. Wu writes in his book about recent research findings:

The research results of Japanese physicians prove that pu-erh tea has anti-cancer effects. This discovery made the tea very popular in Japan. Clinical tests which were carried out jointly by the Medical University of St. Antoine in Paris and the hospital number 1 Medical School Kunming, showed that pu-erh tea has a surprisingly positive effect on fat metabolism. It lowers cholesterol and blood pressure.

In addition, arise in the course of the maturation process in the tea leaves flavones which prevent calcification of arteries.

In the said anti-cancer effect, it is obvious to the particularly pronounced in Pu-erh teas amount of epigallocatechin gallate. These proteins, trace elements, vitamins, and minerals come in a unique combination. From tea quality level of 10 to one, the proportion of valuable substances, however, differs considerably.

In summary, one can say that the investment in tea of higher quality definitely pays off when the present test results are in. You will find a wonderful overview of these results and other research findings in the book by Dr. Wu.

SIX

TEA PREPARATION

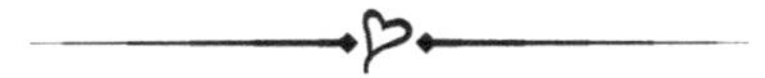

Whether you want to drink pu-erh tea for health reasons or because of enjoyment: It is important that your tea is stored well. Please note that pu-erh tea is a fermented tea, so of course the domestic rests in it can continue to evolve. For this reason, he should not be kept in an airtight Krause. Ideal is an unglazed ceramic vessel.

Unlike other teas, this tea can be stored for a long time. In China teas of different vintages are offered. The whole is comparable with the vintages of fine wines. International finds even teas to more than fifty years in the trade. Stored correctly, the spicy treasures gain over time in terms of quality. Top quality products are even stored much longer. Such teas cost about as much as top wines.

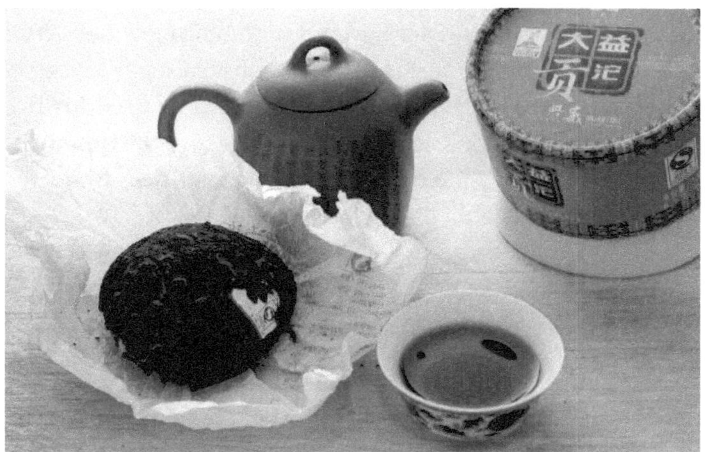

If you purchased the tea in a cake pan, you should replace the blades in use with a pointed object carefully. In China, one uses a special tea knife. With the fine blade, the individual leaves are removed from the cake, without injuring them or breaking them. Broken blades can make the tea bitter.

Tea connoisseurs use a typical Chinese teapot of clay to prepare the tea. Who has no such pot can use an ordinary teapot. The vessel is preheated and swung out with hot water. You can reach the best results with soft, clean water, which was sidelined before cooking.

5 to 20 grams of leaves are then added to the pot and poured over a quarter liter of boiling water, depending on the quality of tea. This first infusion is poured off after a few seconds. It cannot be drunk because it is much too strong and bitter.

Only the second infusion is suitable for pleasure. The now moistened leaves are covered with boiling water. After five to ten seconds, it is poured the tea into a separate vessel (or equal to the cup). The damp leaves can be used for five to ten more infusions. However, the taste and the quality of the ingredients in the first five infusions is best (the first, bitter infusion is not counted).

The tea is drunk slowly and in small sips.

SEVEN

USEFUL APPLICATION RANGES

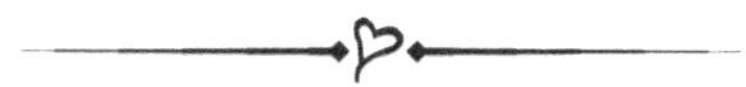

Based on different sources from China - but also the West -, here is a compilation of health ailments, where pu-erh tea is used for. It is strongly advised to seek treatment for all sorts of diseases by a trained person and to carry out all activities in this area only in consultation with a specialist. This also clears you from any possible side effects and interactions with other therapists.

The most common acne occurs during puberty. The skin pores become clogged by excessive sebum production of the skin and leads to inflammation. Similar conditions may occur if the ventilation of the skin with the environment will be affected, for instance by the strong use of cosmetics. Furthermore, acne can be triggered by an unbalanced diet, poisoning and fungal infections in the gut, metabolic disorders, and mental problems.

Due to its composition Pu-erh stimulates the metabolism and thus helps in detoxification and cleansing of the body. Often this secondary disease deprives the foundation.

In addition, the washing with (cold) pu-erh tea and facial steam baths have been proven for skin care. The latter one is steaming tea into a bowl and keeps her head about. Cover both with a towel. The steam opens the pores and cleanses the skin.

Allergies

Pu-erh tea strengthens the immune system and soothes allergic reactions. To stimulate the immune system, the intake of one-liter pu-erh tea is recommended.

Arthritis

Due to its detoxifying effects, metabolism and immune system stimulating effects pu-erh tea reduce arthritic complaints. A combination with a colon cleanse - for example, based on aloe vera - is recommended.

Asthma

Asthma is a chronic respiratory disease. The regular consumption of pu-erh tea strengthens the immune system, which can reduce asthma. In addition, facial steam baths are felt with a decoction of sage and Pu-erh leaves by many stakeholders as soothing. To do this, use both types equally.

Respiratory problems and colds

As it has been said, pu-erh tea reinforces the immune system. Even with pre-existing medical conditions, it can stop several effects. Moreover, it is a proven precautionary measure for a long time to consume in the "cold season" just a few weeks pu-erh tea.

Again, for the treatment of nasal congestion and cough, face steam baths are advisable, as they are described under "asthma".

Flatulence

Flatulence is often caused by spoilage bacteria in the gut. Their formation is favored especially by eating a lot of meat, but also dairy products. Pu-erh tea counteracts here through its purifying and draining power. An ideal complement is the intake of aloe vera.

Increased blood pressure

In traditional Chinese medicine, there is the following recipe: Take equal parts approximately 10 grams of hawthorn, peppermint leaves, and pu-erh tea and pour the mixture with a quarter liter of hot (not boiling) water. Drink it every day one or two cups.

This mixture lowers blood pressure and cholesterol levels. It is even used for weight loss.

Cellulite

Pu-erh tea stimulates the metabolism. Thus, toxins are excreted more rapidly. Also, the rubbing of corresponding points with a rough face cloth, which has been soaked in cold pu-erh tea can help. This promotes blood circulation to the skin, which accelerates the removal of emplaced in fat cells.

In the long term, cellulitis can only be fought by a change in diet and exercise.

Increased cholesterol

See: increased blood pressure

Intestinal infections and constipation

Intestinal infections and constipation can have different causes. Putrefaction bacteria, fungi, but also viruses, retention of Fecaloma and resulting inflammation can trigger diseases. This in turn leads in some cases to auto poisoning of the body as well as to relevant sequelae.

Pu-erh tea has a detoxifying and antibacterial effect. It is like the fluid and mineral loss from successful and stimulates intestinal activity. One to two liters of pu-erh tea are generally a promising idea. A combination with Aloe vera is useful.

Diabetes mellitus

Even for diabetics it is a suitable tea. A good recipe here consists of 50 grams of dried green beans that are even cooked in a liter of water. Subsequently, 5 teaspoons of pu-erh tea and 3 slices of ginger root should be taken. The whole thing should take 5 minutes, then it is strained.

Keep the drink in a sealed vessel and drink it throughout the day. Chinese sources describe it as a sustained improvement in glucose levels after about three months.

Diarrhea

See: intestinal infections

Sleep issues

People with difficulty falling asleep report a very positive effect of the following: just before falling asleep, consume a large cup of hot take pu-erh tea, mixed with a teaspoon of honey dissolved and the juice of half a lemon.

Fever

Fever is in itself a defense reaction of the body to acute infections. The increased body temperature viruses are killed and the immune system strengthened. Pu-erh tea supports this process optimally. You can combine this cure quiet with proven home remedies of vinegar socks up to Wade winding.

Lipid levels in the blood (lipemia)

A study by the Paris St. Antoine Clinic found that can help reduce the levels of blood lipids of patients within one month to thirteen percent when drinking three cups of pu-erh tea per day. In addition, a significant reduction in triglycerides was noted.

Consequences of alcohol consumption

Heike van Braak describes in her book, a study by French scientists. This found that pu-erh tea lowers the alcohol level in the blood. The reason is that pu-erh tea stimulates the activity of the liver, which provides for the reduction of the alcohol.

Hemorrhoids

Grind per 10 grams kelp, pu-erh tea and endive in a mortar and mix the whole with Vaseline. Coat the affected area. In addition, itself recommend a diet adjustment and a colon cleansing.

Hayfever

For the treatment of hayfever, some authors recommend the following recipe: mix a teaspoon of pu-erh tea leaves with about the same amount of finely chopped ginger roots and 10 fresh dandelion leaves. All this is doused with hot water and left to brew ten minutes.

With this, wash the face, nose and eyelids. The substance can be easily massaged. Alternatively, it is possible to use the still steaming tea as a facial steam.

Immunodeficiency

As demonstrated by various scientific studies, pu-erh tea strengthens the immune system. People with immunocompromise problems can use these advantages as a habit to drink a liter of pu-erh tea daily.

Headache / migraine

Cut the rind of (unsprayed) organic orange into small pieces and pour over them boiling with one liter of water. Enter then add a teaspoon of pu-erh tea and 2 teaspoons of honey. Drink the mixture throughout the day.

Liver disorders

Pu-erh tea has a detoxifying and purifying. In addition, it stimulates the metabolism of the liver and kidneys. It makes sense to consume at least 3 large cups pu-erh tea a day.

Stomach discomfort

Stomach discomfort has like most diseases different reasons. Therefore, it is recommended that for every illness you take consultation with a specialist. However, the antibacterial ingredients in Pu-erh teas fight unwanted bacteria in the digestive tract, which the body detoxifies and purifies. The metabolism is positively influenced.

Kidneys and bladder disorders

Kidney and bladder are responsible for detoxification in the body. To function properly, they need plenty of fluids (at least 2 liters per day). Pu-erh tea has a detoxifying and purifying. In addition, it stimulates the metabolism of the liver and kidneys. Sensible drinking at least 3 cups of large pu-erh tea daily is useful.

Edema

Pu-erh tea stimulates the kidney activity. This in turn increases the excretion of water, which promotes the breakdown of blood fluids in tissue columns.

Premenstrual Syndrome (PMS)

Pu-erh tea has a detoxifying effect, which - when consumed regularly - prevents weight gain. It also lightens the mood, thus reducing psychological impairments.

Metabolic disorders

Metabolic disorders cause different diseases that are presented separately in this book. As demonstrated in clinical trials, pu-erh heats tea the metabolism and supports the body optimally for purification, detoxification and also in weight reduction. It is recommended to drink daily 1 to 2 liters of pu-erh tea.

Overweight

See: increased blood pressure

Constipation

See: intestinal infections and constipation

EIGHT

CONTRA INDICATORS

Basically, pu-erh tea is a non-prescription stimulant such as green tea or black tea. People with health issues or intolerances on the mentioned teas should be cautious regarding the quantity and consumption and should consult in any case with the physician of their choice.

As so often in life, the quantity and quality of consumed teas make the difference - in this case between wholesomeness and health damage. If you have any adverse effects, you should consult a doctor you trust.

NINE

SOURCES

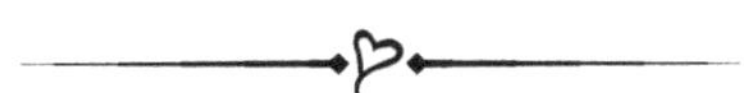

Pu-Erh teas you can buy in most tea shops. Unfortunately, many open mixtures offered, whose quality level and origin are no longer traceable. Also, some Pu-Erh-specialists can be found on the net.

TEN

BIBLIOGRAPHY

- Braunschweig, Ruth von: Pu-Erh-Tee, G & U, 1999
- Greveling, Anne: Pu-Erh-Tee, Urania, 1999
- Grunert, Peter: Pu-erh, das Wundermittel aus Yunnan: Mythen, Legenden und Wahrheiten über einen ungewöhnlichen Tee, Kern, 1999
- Harney, Michael: The Harney & Sons Guide to Tea, Penguin Press, 2008
- Heiß, Mary Lou u. Robert J.: The Tea Enthusiasts Handbook, Ten Speed Press, 2010
- Ling, Wang: Die chinesische Teekultur, 2005, Verlag für fremdsprachige Literatur
- Lübeck, Walter: Pu-Erh-Tee richtig anwenden, Wildpferd, 1999
- Muliar, Doris: Pu-Erh Tee, Falken, 1999
- Oppliger, Peter: Das neue Buch vom grünen Tee, Weltbild, 1999
- Pöhler, Jörg: Gesund mit Pu-Erh-Tee, Droemer, 1999
- Pong, Chan kam: A Glossary of Chinese Puerh Tea, Wushing Books, 2008
- Seifen, Martina: Pu-Erh, Econ, 1999

- Teufl, Cornelia: Gesundheitselixier Grüner Tee, Falken, 1999
- Teusen, Gertrud: Pu-Erh, Kombucha, Ginkgo. Asiatische Wege zur Idealfigur, Bassermann, 1999
- Weilhofer, Dr. Jürgen: PU-ERH – Roter Tee nicht nur Fettkiller, Sanoform, 2000
- Wu, Dr. Li: Fatburner Pu-Erh-Tee. Cholesterin senken mit dem König der chinesischen Tees, Weltbild, 1999
- Van Braak, Heike: Gesund und schlank mit Pu-Erh-Tee – Der Rote Tee aus China, Open Publishing, 2015
- Zittlau, Jörg: Erfolgreich abnehmen mit Pu-erh-Tee, Ludwig, 1999
- Zittlau, Dr. Jörg: Grüner Tee für Gesundheit und Vitalität, Ludwig, 1997

Disclaimer

Introduction

By using this book, you accept this disclaimer in full.

No advice

The book contains information. The information is not advice and should not be treated as such.

No representations or warranties

To the maximum extent permitted by applicable law and subject to section below, we exclude all representations, warranties, undertakings and guarantees relating to the book.

Without prejudice to the generality of the foregoing paragraph, we do not represent, warrant, undertake or guarantee:

- that the information in the book is correct, accurate, complete or non-misleading.

- that the use of the guidance in the book will lead to any particular outcome or result.

Limitations and exclusions of liability

The limitations and exclusions of liability set out in this section and elsewhere in this disclaimer: are subject to section 6 below; and govern all liabilities arising under the disclaimer or in relation to the book, including liabilities arising in contract, in tort (including negligence) and for breach of statutory duty.

We will not be liable to you in respect of any losses arising out of any event or events beyond our reasonable control.

We will not be liable to you in respect of any business losses, including without limitation loss of or damage to profits, income, revenue, use, production, anticipated savings, business, contracts, commercial opportunities or goodwill.

We will not be liable to you in respect of any loss or corruption of any data, database or software.

We will not be liable to you in respect of any special, indirect or consequential loss or damage.

Exceptions

Nothing in this disclaimer shall: limit or exclude our liability for death or personal injury resulting from negligence; limit or exclude our liability for fraud or fraudulent misrepresentation; limit any of our liabilities in any way that is not permitted under applicable law; or exclude any of our liabilities that may not be excluded under applicable law.

Severability

If a section of this disclaimer is determined by any court or other competent authority to be unlawful and/or unenforceable, the other sections of this disclaimer continue in effect.

If any unlawful and/or unenforceable section would be lawful or enforceable if part of it were deleted, that part will be deemed to be deleted, and the rest of the section will continue in effect.

Law and jurisdiction

This disclaimer will be governed by and construed in accordance with Swiss law, and any disputes relating to this disclaimer will be subject to the exclusive jurisdiction of the courts of Switzerland.